# Preface

In a world where childhood obesity has reached alarming proportions, it's clear that traditional approaches are falling short. The urgent need for innovative solutions has never been greater. As we navigate the complex landscape of childhood obesity, it's time to shift our perspective and explore uncharted territories.

Welcome to a journey that transcends the ordinary, a journey that invites you to think beyond the norms and embrace unconventional strategies. This book is a rallying call to challenge the status quo and discover 25 captivating and imaginative ways to address childhood obesity. These are not your run-of-the-mill tactics; they are unique, engaging, and, above all, effective in fostering a generation of healthier, happier children.

Prepare to embark on a voyage that will inspire, inform, and empower. These strategies, born from a fusion of creativity, science, and compassion, hold the potential to reshape the way we approach childhood obesity. Through interactive cooking adventures, nature scavenger hunts, DIY fitness equipment crafts, and more, we will delve into the uncharted waters of prevention, learning, and well-being.

As you turn the pages, consider this your call to action. Each strategy is a blueprint for change, an opportunity to transform not only the lives of children but also the way we view health and wellness. Join us on this unconventional journey, where the possibilities are as limitless as a child's imagination and as impactful as the health of generations to come.

Welcome to "25 Unusual Strategies to Address Childhood Obesity." Get ready to explore, learn, and be inspired. Your journey begins now.

# Introduction

In a world where screens often replace playgrounds and convenience trumps nutritious choices, childhood obesity is a daunting challenge of our time. The battle against this pervasive health issue demands innovative thinking, unorthodox solutions, and a departure from the conventional playbook. Welcome to "25 Creative Ways to Address Childhood Obesity," a journey into a realm where play, imagination, and unconventional strategies take center stage in the fight for a healthier future.

Childhood obesity is not a localized concern; it's a global epidemic that threatens the well-being and vitality of the youngest generation. According to the World Health Organization (WHO), the number of overweight or obese children under the age of five reached an alarming 41 million globally. This statistic is not merely a figure; it's a call to action. It signifies that our traditional approaches, though vital, need augmentation with innovative methods that break free from the confines of routine.

The health implications of childhood obesity are profound and far-reaching, extending well beyond the confines of childhood. From a physical perspective, obese children are more likely to develop chronic conditions like diabetes, cardiovascular diseases, and joint problems, setting the stage for a lifetime of health challenges. Equally concerning are the psychological tolls: low self-esteem, depression, and an increased risk of developing eating disorders can persist into adulthood. Moreover, childhood obesity poses a socioeconomic burden on healthcare systems, diverting resources that could otherwise be invested in preventive measures and quality healthcare. The path forward is not simply about shedding pounds; it's about fostering a holistic shift in our approach to health—one that's built upon innovation and the recognition that one-size-fits-all solutions are no longer sufficient.

As we stand at the intersection of traditional prevention strategies and a changing world, it's evident that a new approach is needed to address childhood obesity. While nutrition education and physical activity promotion remain crucial, they must be complemented by a broader, more imaginative toolkit. The conventional focus on calorie counting and rigid exercise regimens often falls short in capturing the essence of a child's boundless energy and curiosity. It's time to embrace strategies that tap into their innate creativity and zest for life—strategies that blur the lines between play and wellness. "25 Creative Ways to Address Childhood Obesity" introduces a paradigm shift that celebrates innovative thinking, holistic well-being, and personalized approaches. By embracing the power of unconventional ideas and diverse inspirations, we can cultivate a generation of children who not only defy the odds against obesity but also flourish in every aspect of their lives.

As concerned parents, caregivers, educators, and health professionals, we find ourselves at a crossroads, responsible for reshaping the narrative surrounding childhood health. This book is a manifesto for change, an invitation to explore 25 imaginative strategies that challenge the status quo, redefine wellness, and engage children in ways that ignite their passion for a healthy life. Each chapter of this book introduces a distinct approach, offering a glimpse into a world where wellness transcends the scale, and where solutions are as diverse as the children we aim to empower. From transforming household chores into playful adventures to discovering the magic of mindful eating, these unconventional strategies inspire us to rethink our relationship with childhood obesity.

Our journey begins with a simple premise: that the fight against childhood obesity can be both effective and joyful. By coloring outside the lines of tradition, we embrace the spirit of innovation that is so inherently human. We challenge ourselves to seek unconventional inspiration from unlikely sources, to shatter preconceptions, and to foster an environment where every child has the opportunity to thrive.

So, let us embark on this transformative expedition together. Let us explore, imagine, and innovate. As we journey through "25 Creative Ways to Address Childhood Obesity," may we be inspired to rewrite the story of childhood health, one vibrant idea at a time.

# Strategy 1: Cooking Adventures

"Cooking Adventures" are a remarkable and engaging way to foster a genuine appreciation for cooking and nutritious ingredients. Parents should involve their children in the process of creating their own meals to nurture their health and ignite a lifelong passion for wholesome living.

## Exploring the Concept

At the heart of Cooking Adventures lies the understanding that when children participate in preparing their meals, they form a deeper connection with the food they eat. This connection transcends the superficial act of consumption, transforming meals into a canvas for creativity, learning, and exploration. This strategy encourages them to actively engage with the ingredients, understand their origins, and make conscious choices about what they put on their plates.

## The Adventure Unveiled

Imagine a group of young explorers gathering around a kitchen table, armed with aprons and curiosity. Guided by an adult or caregiver, they embark on an adventure to create a nutritious meal from scratch. From selecting fresh vegetables at the market to measuring ingredients with colorful measuring cups, each step is an opportunity for discovery.

**Step 1: Exploration and Selection:** The adventure begins with a trip to the local farmer's market or grocery store. Children are encouraged to pick out ingredients for a specific dish, introducing them to the vibrant world of fruits, vegetables, and whole grains. This hands-on experience allows them to touch, smell, and learn about different ingredients.

**Step 2: Hands-On Preparation:** Back in the kitchen, children roll up their sleeves and dive into the culinary process. They wash, chop, and mix ingredients, experiencing the transformation of raw materials into a delicious meal. This tactile experience engages their senses, making the connection between whole foods and the nourishment they provide.

**Step 3: Creative Culinary Exploration:** As the cooking adventure unfolds, children are encouraged to experiment with flavors. They add herbs, spices, and other seasonings, discovering the alchemy that turns simple ingredients into delectable dishes. This creative freedom not only makes cooking enjoyable but also empowers children to tailor their meals to their taste preferences.

**Step 4: Savoring the Fruits of Labor:** Finally, the cooking adventure culminates in a shared meal. Children proudly present their creations to family and friends, relishing the satisfaction of having contributed to the table. This communal experience reinforces the value of cooking as a way to bring people together and create positive associations with healthy eating.

## Preventing Childhood Obesity

Cooking Adventures hold tremendous potential in preventing childhood obesity through several key mechanisms:

**Connection with Nutritious Foods:** When children actively engage in preparing meals, they develop a firsthand understanding of the nutritional value of ingredients. This awareness lays the groundwork for making healthier food choices in the future.

**Empowerment and Education:** Cooking Adventures empower children to make informed decisions about their diet. By learning about ingredients, portion sizes, and cooking methods, they gain skills that contribute to lifelong healthy eating habits.

**Diverse Palate Development:** Experimentation with different flavors and ingredients broadens children's palates, making them more receptive to a variety of foods. This openness to diverse options reduces the likelihood of unhealthy eating patterns.

**Positive Associations with Food:** Cooking Adventures create positive emotional connections with food, emphasizing the joy of preparing and sharing meals. Such positive associations help counteract negative emotional eating habits.

**Family Engagement:** Cooking Adventures foster family bonding, encouraging children to connect with their caregivers and peers over shared culinary experiences. This environment promotes a supportive foundation for healthy living.

In essence, the "Cooking Adventures" strategy is a celebration of the art of cooking and the science of nutrition. It's a journey that guides children toward a deeper understanding of food, cultivating a lifelong love for culinary exploration. By sowing the seeds of appreciation for cooking and nutritious ingredients, we foster health, resilience, and wellbeing that flourish long into adulthood.

# Strategy 2: Active Storytelling

In the realm of childhood obesity prevention, imagination and movement unite in a powerful strategy known as "Active Storytelling." This innovative approach captivates young minds while inspiring them to embrace an active lifestyle by infusing storytelling with physical activities. The pages of books come alive, and characters' journeys become invitations for children to embark on their own adventures of motion and exploration.

Unveiling Active Storytelling: Imagine a world where storytelling isn't confined to words on a page but extends to the realm of movement and action. Through "Active Storytelling," children are introduced to narratives that seamlessly integrate physical activities into the plot. As characters in the story jump, dance, climb, and run, children mirror these actions, transforming sedentary reading time into a dynamic, engaging experience.

## Crafting Enchanted Adventures

Picture a group of children gathered in a circle, eager to embark on an adventure guided by a storyteller. The tale begins with vivid descriptions of characters' activities: heroes climbing mountains, fairies leaping over streams, and explorers racing against the wind. With each plot twist, children mimic the characters' movements, embodying the story's energy and enthusiasm.

**Example: The Great Forest Quest:** In "The Great Forest Quest," young readers journey alongside Alex, a brave adventurer exploring a magical forest. As the story unfolds, Alex encounters friendly creatures who challenge them to various tasks. When a wise owl challenges Alex to balance on one foot like a graceful flamingo, children in the audience mirror the action. When Alex races a squirrel through a maze of trees, young listeners mimic the running, turning, and dodging described in the narrative.

## Preventing Childhood Obesity Through Active Imagination

"Active Storytelling" boasts a myriad of benefits that contribute to preventing childhood obesity:

**Embodied Learning**: By physically engaging with stories, children absorb the joy of movement organically. Active participation helps reinforce the concept that exercise can be fun and exhilarating.

**Role Modeling**: Characters in active stories become role models for healthy behavior. As children connect with these characters, they internalize the idea that being active is a positive and integral part of life.

**Cognitive Engagement**: Combining physical actions with storytelling enhances cognitive engagement. Children's brains light up as they coordinate movements with the narrative, promoting cognitive development alongside physical activity.

**Creating Active Habits**: Active Storytelling instills the habit of movement at a young age. This foundation can help children carry forward a positive relationship with exercise into adolescence and adulthood.

## Inclusivity and Joy

Active Storytelling is inclusive, accommodating varying abilities and levels of physical fitness. It creates a joyful atmosphere where children of all backgrounds can participate and thrive.

Through "Active Storytelling," children not only embark on imaginary journeys but embark on journeys of self-discovery and empowerment. As they mimic characters' movements, they explore the boundless potential of their own bodies. By weaving movement seamlessly into the fabric of stories, we guide children toward the path of an active, healthy lifestyle—one where physical activity is celebrated as a magical adventure in its own right.

# Strategy 3: Community Garden Projects

Amid the concrete jungles of modern life, an oasis of health, connection, and education blooms through the strategy of "Community Garden Projects." This innovative approach invites children to roll up their sleeves and become stewards of the earth. They engage in hands-on gardening experiences that foster an appreciation for fresh produce, nurture physical activity, and cultivate a sense of community.

**Sowing the Seeds of Connection:** Picture a piece of unused land transformed into a vibrant community garden—a place where children and families gather to plant, nurture, and reap the rewards of their efforts. Community Garden Projects introduce children to the world of gardening, encouraging them to dig, plant, water, and harvest alongside their peers and mentors.

## The Gardening Journey

In the heart of the community garden, children embark on a journey that is both educational and transformative. They learn about soil health, the seasons, the life cycles of plants, and the intricate dance of pollinators. With each turn of the soil, they gain an understanding of the intimate relationship between nature's rhythms and the food on their plates.

**The Bountiful Harvest:** As the garden flourishes, children experience the thrill of watching their efforts come to fruition. They pick ripe tomatoes, pluck fragrant herbs, and harvest colorful vegetables. These moments of triumph inspire not only a sense of accomplishment but also a profound appreciation for the fruits of nature's labor.

## Cultivating Health and Preventing Obesity

"Community Garden Projects" holds immense potential in preventing childhood obesity by promoting healthy behaviors:

**Hands-On Education:** Children gain practical knowledge about where food comes from, deepening their connection to fresh, whole foods and encouraging them to make healthier choices.

**Physical Activity:** Gardening is inherently physical, involving digging, planting, weeding, and more. This hands-on engagement promotes physical activity without feeling like exercise, helping to combat sedentary habits.

**Nutritional Awareness:** As children witness the growth of vegetables and herbs, they develop a heightened awareness of the nutritional value of different foods. This awareness influences their food choices beyond the garden.

**Empowerment:** Through their contributions to the garden's success, children experience a sense of empowerment and ownership over their health and the health of their community.

**Community Building:** Community Garden Projects create spaces for families, neighbors, and children to come together, fostering social connections and a sense of belonging.

## Growing Healthy Futures

In the nurturing embrace of a community garden, children discover the joys of working with the earth, witnessing the magic of growth, and reaping the rewards of their labor. Community Garden Projects not only teach children about horticulture but also about life's interconnectedness—the delicate balance of nature and our role in preserving it. As they engage in planting and nurturing, they are simultaneously planting the seeds of a healthier future—one where the earth's bounty becomes a source of nourishment, learning, and joy. Through these projects, we celebrate not just the harvest of fresh produce, but the harvest of vibrant health and thriving communities.

# Strategy 4: Artistic Food Creations

In the quest to address childhood obesity, the strategy of "Artistic Food Creations" offers a delightful twist that fuses imagination with nutrition. By inviting children to turn their meals into captivating works of art, this innovative approach transforms the act of eating into a joyful exploration of color, texture, and creativity.

Unleashing Culinary Creativity: Imagine a plate transformed into a canvas and a meal into a masterpiece. "Artistic Food Creations" encourages children to look at their dishes in a new light, viewing each ingredient as a vibrant hue in their artistic palette. By arranging fruits, vegetables, and other wholesome ingredients into playful shapes, patterns, and scenes, children are drawn into a world where nourishment is as much about visual pleasure as it is about sustenance.

## The Art of Nourishment

In the heart of this strategy, children become culinary artists, wielding their utensils as brushes and their plates as canvases. Carrots transform into sunshine rays, broccoli morphs into trees, and whole grain bread becomes the foundation for edible sculptures. Every meal becomes an opportunity for creative expression, an invitation to infuse healthy eating with imaginative flair.

**Example: The Garden Patch Salad:** Imagine a vibrant salad as an artistic canvas. A bed of lettuce forms the base, while tomatoes are arranged to resemble a row of colorful flowers. Cucumber slices become leaves, and a drizzle of yogurt dressing adds a touch of whimsy, mimicking a winding garden path. As children assemble their garden patch salad, they engage not only with their sense of taste but also with their innate creativity.

**Example: The Rainbow Toast Delight**: Imagine a morning scene at the breakfast table where "Artistic Food Creations" take center stage. A slice of whole-grain toast becomes the canvas for a vibrant masterpiece. Children are invited to explore the colors of the rainbow using an array of nutritious toppings. Here's how the transformation unfolds:

**Red**: A spread of antioxidant-rich strawberry jam forms the first layer, resembling the dawn of a colorful day.

**Orange**: Slices of ripe and juicy orange, arranged in a circular pattern, mimic the rising sun and infuse the toast with a burst of citrus flavor.

**Yellow**: A drizzle of honey or a sprinkle of golden chia seeds represents the radiant warmth of sunlight.

**Green**: Fresh avocado slices, carefully placed in a leafy pattern, evoke the tranquility of nature and offer healthy fats.

**Blue**: A dollop of blueberry yogurt or a scattering of blueberries introduces a cool, calming touch reminiscent of clear skies.

**Purple**: A final touch of sliced grapes or a dash of antioxidant-packed acai powder represents the magical hues of dusk.

As children assemble their rainbow toast, they explore the colorful spectrum of fruits, seeds, and spreads, enhancing their understanding of various nutrients and their benefits. With each bite, they experience a symphony of flavors, textures, and colors that fuel both their bodies and their creative spirits.

The Rainbow Toast Delight exemplifies how "Artistic Food Creations" can transform a simple meal into a captivating visual and sensory experience. By merging artistic expression with nutritional exploration, children not only develop a more profound connection to the foods they eat but also cultivate a positive relationship with healthy choices. This approach encourages them to see food as an opportunity for self-expression and nourishment, contributing to their overall well-being and, ultimately, supporting the prevention of childhood obesity.

## Promoting Healthy Eating and Preventing Obesity

"Artistic Food Creations" holds several key benefits in the prevention of childhood obesity:

**Engaging Presentation:** By transforming meals into visually appealing creations, children are drawn to healthier options with a sense of excitement and curiosity.

**Nutritional Awareness:** As children experiment with arranging different food items, they gain an understanding of the nutritional value of each ingredient, fostering mindful eating habits.

**Culinary Exploration:** Artistic Food Creations encourage children to explore a diverse range of foods and flavors, expanding their palate and reducing the risk of food monotony.

**Positive Associations:** By associating healthy foods with creativity and enjoyment, children develop positive attitudes toward nutritious options, mitigating the allure of less healthy alternatives.

**Family Bonding:** Preparing and enjoying artistic meals together can become a family activity, fostering shared experiences and conversations about healthy eating.

## Crafting a Nutritional Masterpiece

In the canvas of "Artistic Food Creations," the boundaries between nutrition and creativity blur. This strategy elevates meals from mere sustenance to nourishment for the body and soul. As children design, assemble, and delight in their edible creations, they forge a profound connection between art and health, imagination and wellness. In this vibrant world, food becomes a medium for self-expression and exploration, cultivating not only healthy eating habits but also a lifelong love for culinary ingenuity.

# Strategy 5: Dance and Movement Play - Infusing Joyful Activity into Playtime

In the spirited world of childhood, where imagination knows no bounds, "Dance and Movement Play" is a dynamic strategy that intertwines physical activity with pure delight. By seamlessly integrating dance and movement challenges into playtime, this approach transforms exercise into a lively adventure, inviting children to revel in the joy of movement while nurturing their bodies.

**The Dance of Play and Health:** Imagine a playground transformed into a stage where every swing, hop, and skip becomes part of an enchanting dance. "Dance and Movement Play" introduces children to the notion that physical activity is not a chore but a joyful rhythm that dances to the beat of their hearts. Through creative movement challenges and games, children are encouraged to explore their bodies' capabilities and celebrate the sheer exhilaration of being active.

## Embracing Movement Adventures

In the heart of this strategy lies a world of imaginative movement adventures. Picture children becoming pirates on a treasure hunt, their movements mirroring the swaying of the ship as they climb ladders, leap over "waves," and navigate through imaginary obstacles. Alternatively, envision them as jungle explorers, crawling beneath "branches," jumping over "rivers," and imitating the calls of wild animals. Each movement is an invitation for laughter, creativity, and the sheer fun of being in motion.

Example: The Freeze Dance Challenge: Imagine a play area transformed into a dance floor where music sets the tempo for the game. In the "Freeze Dance Challenge," children groove to the rhythm, allowing their bodies to flow freely. When the music suddenly stops, they strike a pose, capturing the movement in a freeze frame. As the music resumes, they seamlessly transition back into dancing, celebrating both the movement and the anticipation of the freeze.

## Promoting Active Joy and Preventing Obesity

"Dance and Movement Play" offers a range of benefits in the prevention of childhood obesity:

**Enjoyable Physical Activity**: By infusing playtime with dance and movement, children discover the pleasure of staying active, redefining physical exercise as a source of enjoyment.

**Cardiovascular Health**: Dance and movement activities elevate heart rates, promoting cardiovascular fitness and overall well-being.

**Motor Skills**: Creative movement challenges enhance coordination, balance, and agility, crucial for healthy physical development.

**Social Interaction**: Movement games foster social connections as children engage in cooperative play, developing communication and teamwork skills.

**Boosting Confidence**: Movement challenges encourage self-expression and body awareness, promoting a positive body image and boosting self-confidence.

## In the Dance of Life

In the realm of "Dance and Movement Play," the playground becomes a stage, and physical activity becomes a joyful dance. This strategy champions the idea that exercise is not a duty but an expression of vitality and exuberance. By engaging in playful movement challenges, children discover that being active can be as natural as laughter, as instinctive as play, and as nourishing as friendship. As they embrace the dance of life, they dance toward a future filled with health, happiness, and a deep appreciation for the magic of movement.

# Strategy 6: Superhero Training Camp

Amidst the realms of fantasy and reality, the "Superhero Training Camp" is an ingenious strategy that ignites the spark of heroism while nurturing a love for physical activity. By designing imaginative training activities inspired by superheroes, this approach transforms exercise into a thrilling adventure, allowing children to become the heroes of their own stories.

**The Call to Heroic Play:** Imagine a world where children don capes and embark on epic quests to save the day. The "Superhero Training Camp" takes children on an exhilarating journey, where they transform into caped crusaders, armored knights, or mighty protectors, all while engaging in exercises that seamlessly blend play and physical activity.

## Creating Heroic Challenges

At the core of this strategy lies a series of challenges that combine superhero-inspired actions with exercises. Picture children leaping over "buildings" (cones), crawling through "tunnels" (playground equipment), and scaling "walls" (climbing structures). Each challenge is infused with imaginative storytelling, inviting children to use their bodies to conquer obstacles and complete heroic feats.

Example: The Speedster Dash: Imagine a challenge inspired by the speed of the fastest superheroes. Children line up at the starting line, donning their superhero capes. As an enthusiastic leader narrates the tale, they sprint across the "city," zigzagging between cones that represent obstacles, and racing against the clock. The finish line represents a victorious moment, where each child's speedster powers are celebrated with cheers and applause.

## Promoting Heroic Health and Preventing Obesity

The "Superhero Training Camp" holds a range of benefits in the prevention of childhood obesity:

**Engagement Through Imagination:** By merging play and physical activity with imaginative superhero roles, children are motivated to stay active in a way that sparks their creativity.

**Full-Body Exercise:** Superhero challenges involve a variety of movements, promoting holistic physical development and cardiovascular fitness.

**Motor Skills Enhancement:** As children crawl, leap, and run through challenges, their motor skills and coordination are honed.

**Self-Esteem Boost:** The role of a hero fosters self-confidence, empowering children to overcome challenges and celebrate their accomplishments.

**Social Bonding:** Superhero challenges encourage teamwork, cooperation, and camaraderie as children unite in their quest to save the day.

## In the Realm of Heroes

In the enchanting landscape of the "Superhero Training Camp," children don't just exercise; they embody the spirit of heroism and adventure. Through creative challenges and imaginative storytelling, they learn that being active isn't merely a task but a heroic endeavor. As they leap, run, and conquer, they become the champions of their own stories, carrying the lessons of health, courage, and imagination into every aspect of their lives. In this world, fitness isn't just a goal—it's a heroic journey toward strength, vitality, and the triumphant pursuit of well-being.

# Strategy 7: Healthy Habit Rewards

The strategy of "Healthy Habit Rewards" is a delightful approach that embraces positive reinforcement without relying on traditional food-based incentives. By celebrating children's healthy choices with non-food rewards like stickers, badges, or small toys, this strategy transforms the path to wellness into a journey filled with excitement, encouragement, and empowerment.

**The Joy of Non-Food Rewards:** Imagine a world where healthy choices are celebrated not with sugary treats, but with colorful stickers, shiny badges, or intriguing small toys. "Healthy Habit Rewards" introduces children to the idea that making positive lifestyle choices comes with its own set of treasures—rewards that spark joy without compromising their health.

## Celebrating Small Triumphs

At the heart of this strategy lies the celebration of everyday victories. Whether a child chooses a piece of fruit over a sugary snack or opts for water instead of a sugary drink, these choices are acknowledged and celebrated through tangible rewards. The act of collecting stickers, earning badges, or receiving small toys becomes a powerful motivator that encourages children to persistently embrace healthy habits.

**Example: The Sticker Challenge:** Imagine a sticker chart displayed prominently in a communal area. Each time a child makes a healthy choice—for instance, opting for a balanced meal or engaging in physical activity—they receive a sticker to place on their chart. As the chart fills up with stickers, children experience a sense of accomplishment and anticipation. When they reach a predetermined goal, they receive a special badge or small toy—a tangible symbol of their dedication to their well-being.

## Promoting Positive Choices and Preventing Obesity

"Healthy Habit Rewards" offers a range of benefits in the prevention of childhood obesity:

**Positive Reinforcement**: Non-food rewards create positive associations with healthy choices, reinforcing the notion that well-being is its own reward.

**Motivation**: The prospect of earning stickers, badges, or small toys encourages children to make healthy decisions consistently.

**Ownership and Empowerment**: Children take charge of their health journey, feeling empowered by the choices they make and the rewards they earn.

**Healthy Habits Formation**: Consistently celebrating small triumphs fosters the establishment of lasting healthy habits.

**Family Engagement**: Families can participate in the reward system, fostering a supportive environment that champions well-being.

## Collecting Moments of Triumph

In the world of "Healthy Habit Rewards," every choice becomes an opportunity for celebration, every small triumph a chance to earn a badge of honor. By transforming the act of making healthy choices into a game of rewards and recognition, we embark on a journey that promotes self-care, motivation, and the cultivation of lifelong well-being. As children collect stickers, badges, and tokens of their achievements, they also collect moments of pride, resilience, and the knowledge that their health is a precious gift to be treasured.

# Strategy 8: Nutrition and Fitness Gaming

In the era of technology, the "Nutrition and Fitness Gaming" strategy emerges as a clever fusion of virtual engagement and real-world health. By introducing video games that not only entertain but also promote healthy eating and physical activity, this approach transforms screen time into a gateway for wellness, seamlessly integrating fun and well-being.

**The Power of Virtual Play**: Imagine a world where video games aren't just a source of entertainment but also a catalyst for healthy habits. "Nutrition and Fitness Gaming" invites children into virtual realms where they embark on adventures that align with their real-world health goals. Through interactive gameplay, children are motivated to make nutritious choices and engage in physical activity in order to advance in the game.

## Creating Health-Promoting Adventures

At the core of this strategy lies a collection of video games specifically designed to encourage healthy behaviors. Picture a game where players guide a character through a vibrant landscape, collecting virtual fruits and vegetables that contribute to their in-game vitality. Another game might challenge players to complete physical movements that correspond to on-screen prompts, fostering real-world physical activity while progressing in the game.

**Example: The Superfood Quest**: Imagine a game where players embark on a Superfood Quest to restore health to a fictional kingdom. In this adventure, players journey through lush landscapes, collecting virtual fruits and vegetables to empower their character. Each nutritious choice enhances the character's abilities and advances the storyline. To make the experience interactive, the game incorporates motion-based controls, encouraging players to perform physical activities like jumping, squatting, and stretching to activate in-game actions.

## Promoting Health-Packed Play and Preventing Obesity

"Nutrition and Fitness Gaming" offers a range of benefits in the prevention of childhood obesity:

**Engagement and Learning:** Through interactive gameplay, children learn about the nutritional value of foods and the importance of physical activity in an engaging and memorable way.

**Incentivizing Healthy Choices:** Virtual rewards and progress in the game become incentives for making positive lifestyle choices in the real world.

**Motor Skill Enhancement:** Games that incorporate physical movements enhance coordination, balance, and motor skills.

**Technological Integration:** This strategy capitalizes on technology's appeal to engage children in health-promoting behaviors.

**Positive Attitudes:** By associating wellness with entertainment, children develop positive attitudes toward nutrition and physical activity.

## Embarking on Virtual Wellness Quests

In the immersive realm of "Nutrition and Fitness Gaming," children don't just play games—they embark on quests for vitality, strength, and well-being. This strategy redefines screen time by leveraging technology as a tool to inspire and empower healthy choices. As children navigate virtual landscapes, they also navigate a path to lifelong health, making meaningful connections between their digital adventures and the real-world pursuit of wellness. In this virtual realm, play is infused with purpose, and every achievement is a step toward a healthier, happier future.

# Strategy 9: Family Fit Challenges

"Family Fit Challenges" is a captivating strategy that intertwines physical activity with cherished family moments. By involving the entire family in fitness challenges or obstacle courses, this approach transforms exercise into a joyful adventure, fostering togetherness, laughter, and a collective commitment to well-being.

**The Power of Family Unity:** Imagine a scenario where the entire family gathers, united by a common goal—to embark on fitness challenges and obstacle courses that strengthen not only their bodies but also their bonds. "Family Fit Challenges" embraces the idea that wellness is not an individual pursuit but a shared journey that thrives when experienced together.

## Creating Fitness Adventures

At the core of this strategy lies the creation of interactive fitness challenges that every family member can partake in. Picture a relay race in the backyard, where each family member takes on a leg of the course, from running and jumping to hopping and crawling. Another challenge might involve creating an obstacle course using household items, encouraging family members to engage in a variety of movements while navigating the course.

**Example: The Amazing Family Race**: Imagine a playful twist on the traditional treasure hunt—the "Amazing Family Race." In this challenge, families work together to decipher clues that lead them to different locations in the neighborhood or around the house. At each stop, they encounter a physical activity challenge that must be completed before moving on to the next clue. These challenges could include jumping jacks, squats, partner yoga poses, or even impromptu dance-offs.

## Promoting Bonding and Preventing Obesity

"Family Fit Challenges" offers a range of benefits beyond physical health:

**Quality Time:** Engaging in fitness challenges fosters precious moments of connection and interaction among family members.

**Positive Role Modeling:** Children witness their parents' commitment to health, creating a strong foundation for their own healthy habits.

**Laughter and Joy:** Shared challenges create opportunities for laughter, joy, and shared memories that reinforce the positive aspects of physical activity.

**Teamwork and Communication:** Collaborative challenges enhance teamwork skills and communication within the family unit.

**Healthy Lifestyle Culture:** Regular family fitness challenges contribute to the cultivation of a wellness-focused family culture.

## Uniting in Wellness Adventures

In the enchanting world of "Family Fit Challenges," the playground extends beyond the physical realm. Families bond, laugh, and sweat together, not just as individuals but as a united force committed to health and happiness. This strategy transforms exercise into a celebration of shared achievements, and fitness into a conduit for family togetherness. As families navigate obstacle courses, complete challenges, and celebrate victories, they forge a stronger bond while building a legacy of well-being that echoes through generations. In this adventure, the family unit becomes a source of strength, joy, and the unbreakable ties that lead to a life well-lived.

# Strategy 10: Digital Device Swap

In the landscape where technology reigns supreme, the "Digital Device Swap" strategy emerges as a clever method to transition screen time into active playtime. By introducing a system that encourages children to exchange their digital device usage for engaging in physical activities, this approach transforms sedentary hours into moments of movement, play, and discovery.

**The Balancing Act:** Imagine a world where children learn to strike a harmonious balance between screen time and active exploration. The "Digital Device Swap" strategy empowers children to recognize that every moment spent engaged in physical activity is a step toward both well-being and enjoyment.

## Trading Screens for Adventures

At the heart of this strategy is a structured system that prompts children to trade screen time for active playtime. Picture a chart or calendar where children log the time they spend engaged in physical activities. For every designated period of activity, they earn credits that can be exchanged for limited screen time, encouraging them to be active before they immerse themselves in digital entertainment.

**Example: The Adventure Exchange:** Imagine a family implementing the "Adventure Exchange" system. For every hour of outdoor play, a child earns a digital device credit that can be redeemed for screen time. The accumulated credits create a sense of achievement and anticipation, making screen time a reward for the efforts invested in active play.

## Promoting Balanced Engagement and Preventing Obesity

"Digital Device Swap" holds several advantages in the context of childhood obesity prevention:

**Active Lifestyle Cultivation**: Children learn to associate physical activity with a reward, fostering a habit of engaging in movement as a joyful endeavor.

**Mindful Screen Time**: The system encourages children to make conscious decisions about screen time, creating awareness around balancing digital engagement with real-world experiences.

**Physical Activity Integration**: Screen time is transformed into a catalyst for active play, ensuring that children don't remain sedentary for extended periods.

**Family Participation:** Families can participate together, reinforcing a collective commitment to wellness and positive technology use.

**Ownership of Choices:** Children learn that they have control over their screen time and that their active participation can lead to rewarding experiences.

## Trading Time for Enriching Moments

In the realm of "Digital Device Swap," time becomes a currency for enriching experiences. This strategy empowers children to make informed decisions about their use of technology while encouraging them to embrace the joys of active play. As they trade screen time for outdoor adventures, games, or imaginative activities, they learn that time invested in movement yields rewards that extend far beyond the screen—a world of vitality, fun, and the vibrant pursuit of well-being.

# Strategy 11: Mindful Eating Exercises

Amidst the rush of modern life, the "Mindful Eating Exercises" strategy emerges as a calming approach that encourages children to forge a mindful relationship with food. By introducing mindful eating techniques that help children connect with their hunger and fullness cues, this approach transforms mealtime into a moment of presence, appreciation, and self-awareness.

The Art of Mindful Eating: Imagine a world where children learn to savor every bite, appreciating the colors, textures, and flavors of their meals. "Mindful Eating Exercises" invite children to slow down, engage their senses, and develop a deeper connection with the nourishment they receive.

## Cultivating Presence at Meals

At the core of this strategy are exercises that teach children to engage with their meals in a mindful manner. Picture a moment where children close their eyes, take a few deep breaths, and engage their senses before eating. They observe the colors, smells, and textures of their food, noticing the sensations of hunger and the subtle cues of fullness that arise as they eat.

**Example: The Savoring Ritual:** Imagine a "savoring ritual" before a meal. Children are guided to hold a piece of their food—a slice of fruit, a vegetable, or a small bite of a meal—in their hand. They are encouraged to observe it closely, noticing its color, shape, and texture. Then, they take a moment to inhale its aroma. As they take their first bite, they focus on the flavors that unfold, savoring each sensation and chewing slowly. This ritual invites children to engage fully with their food and the experience of eating.

## Promoting Mindful Eating and Preventing Obesity

"Mindful Eating Exercises" offer a range of benefits for the prevention of childhood obesity:

**Awareness of Hunger and Fullness:** Children develop a heightened awareness of their body's signals of hunger and fullness, leading to more balanced eating habits.

**Reduced Overeating:** Mindful eating encourages children to eat at a pace that allows them to recognize when they are comfortably full, reducing the likelihood of overeating.

**Appreciation of Food:** By focusing on the sensory aspects of eating, children develop a greater appreciation for the taste and texture of their food.

**Mind-Body Connection:** Mindful eating exercises foster a stronger mind-body connection, enabling children to make more conscious and nourishing food choices.

**Healthy Relationship with Food:** Children learn to view food as nourishment and enjoyment, rather than as a source of emotional comfort or reward.

## Savoring Every Nourishing Moment

In the realm of "Mindful Eating Exercises," mealtime becomes a sanctuary of presence and connection. This strategy invites children to embark on a journey of self-discovery and self-care as they learn to listen to their bodies and savor the nourishing moments that food brings. As children engage with their senses, they cultivate a deeper appreciation for the gift of sustenance and the mindful path to health and well-being.

# Strategy 12: Adventure Day Outings

In the embrace of the great outdoors, the "Adventure Day Outings" strategy comes to life, inviting children to embark on thrilling escapades that fuse exploration with physical activity. By orchestrating outings that involve hiking, geocaching, rock climbing, and more, this approach transforms leisure time into an opportunity for adventure, learning, and vibrant well-being.

**The Wilderness as Playground:** Imagine a world where the vast expanse of nature becomes a canvas for active exploration. "Adventure Day Outings" beckon families to venture into the wilderness, where every trail, rock face, and hidden treasure becomes an invitation to move, discover, and connect with the natural world.

## Crafting Active Expeditions

At the heart of this strategy lies the orchestration of day outings that infuse physical activity with the thrill of adventure. Picture a hike through a scenic trail, where children engage in a natural scavenger hunt for leaves, rocks, or interesting flora and fauna. Alternatively, envision a day of geocaching, where families follow GPS coordinates to uncover hidden treasures, engaging in playful movement along the way.

**Example: The Rock Climbing Quest:** Imagine a family adventure to a local rock climbing destination. Children learn the art of scaling rock faces under the guidance of experienced instructors. The journey combines physical exertion with strategic planning, as children navigate routes that challenge their strength, balance, and problem-solving skills. As they reach the summit, they are rewarded not just with a sense of achievement, but with breathtaking views that remind them of the beauty of the natural world.

## Promoting Active Exploration and Preventing Obesity

"Adventure Day Outings" hold numerous advantages in the realm of childhood obesity prevention:

**Physical Engagement:** Outdoor activities involve a variety of movements that engage muscles, promote cardiovascular health, and encourage active play.

**Nature Connection:** Exploring the outdoors fosters a connection to nature, nurturing a sense of wonder and curiosity that supports a healthy lifestyle.

**Variety and Excitement:** Adventure outings introduce children to new activities, sparking enthusiasm for physical activity beyond traditional exercises.

**Life Skills:** Activities like geocaching and rock climbing enhance problem-solving, teamwork, and resilience, fostering holistic development.

**Positive Memories:** Adventure outings create enduring memories that associate physical activity with joy, excitement, and the thrill of exploration.

## Venturing into the Heart of Nature's Playground

In the realm of "Adventure Day Outings," nature becomes both a sanctuary and a playground—a realm of enchantment waiting to be discovered. This strategy encourages families to embark on expeditions that unite physical activity with the thrill of exploration, offering children the chance to witness the beauty of the world and the power of their own bodies. As they hike, climb, and explore, they cultivate a profound connection to the natural world and an unyielding love for the adventures that lead to a life filled with vitality and awe.

# Strategy 13: Health-Themed Craft Projects

In the realm of artistic exploration, the "Health-Themed Craft Projects" strategy emerges as a dynamic approach that intertwines creativity with the principles of health, nutrition, and physical activity. By engaging children in crafting projects that celebrate well-being, this strategy transforms artistic expression into a vibrant medium for learning, understanding, and embracing a holistic approach to health.

**The Canvas of Wellness:** Imagine a world where art becomes a conduit for understanding the importance of health and well-being. "Health-Themed Craft Projects" invite children to paint, glue, sculpt, and create, using their imagination to bring health-related concepts to life.

## Crafting Creative Connections

At the core of this strategy lies the creation of craft projects that highlight various aspects of health, nutrition, and physical activity. Picture children designing posters that showcase the food groups, sculpting models of the human body to learn about anatomy, or even crafting a healthy food-themed board game that promotes learning through play.

**Example: The Nutrient Collage:** Imagine a crafting project where children create a "Nutrient Collage." Armed with magazines, scissors, and glue, children scour the pages for images of different foods representing various nutrients. They cut out fruits, vegetables, grains, proteins, and dairy products and arrange them on a poster board. As they assemble their collage, they learn about the importance of a balanced diet and the role different nutrients play in their health.

## Promoting Creative Learning and Preventing Obesity

"Health-Themed Craft Projects" offer a range of advantages for childhood obesity prevention:

**Visual Learning:** Crafting projects make health-related concepts tangible and visually engaging, fostering a deeper understanding of wellness.

**Interactive Exploration:** Hands-on projects encourage children to explore health topics in a playful, interactive, and memorable way.

**Artistic Expression:** Children's creativity is celebrated as they transform health-related information into beautiful, meaningful art.

**Educational Reinforcement:** Craft projects reinforce lessons learned about health, nutrition, and physical activity in a creative and imaginative manner.

**Family Engagement:** Craft projects can become family activities, encouraging open discussions about health and well-being.

## Crafting a Canvas of Well-Being

In the world of "Health-Themed Craft Projects," creativity knows no bounds, and the canvas becomes a realm for exploring, learning, and understanding health in all its dimensions. This strategy invites children to use their artistic talents to dive into wellness, nurturing a connection between their creativity and their journey toward a healthier life. As they paint, glue, and shape their way to understanding, they also paint a picture of a future filled with vitality, knowledge, and a passion for embracing well-being in every aspect of their lives.

# Strategy 14: Wellness Journaling

In the realm of self-discovery and introspection, the "Wellness Journaling" strategy emerges as a powerful tool that empowers children to take charge of their health journey. By encouraging children to keep journals tracking their activity levels, food choices, and emotions, this approach transforms writing into a transformative practice that promotes self-awareness, mindful choices, and holistic well-being.

**The Blank Pages of Possibility:** Imagine a world where the pages of a journal become a canvas for self-reflection, growth, and well-being. "Wellness Journaling" invites children to pick up their pens and embark on a journey of introspection and understanding.

## Cultivating Mindful Practices

At the heart of this strategy lies the practice of journaling to track various aspects of health. Picture children jotting down notes about their physical activities, recording the foods they eat, and capturing their emotions and thoughts related to their well-being journey.

**Example: The Daily Wellness Log:** Imagine children keeping a "Daily Wellness Log" in their journals. They write about their physical activities for the day, whether it's walking, playing a sport, or dancing. They record the meals and snacks they eat, paying attention to portion sizes and the balance of nutrients. They also have a section to express their feelings, reflecting on how their activities and food choices make them feel physically and emotionally.

## Promoting Self-Awareness and Preventing Obesity

"Wellness Journaling" offers a range of advantages in the prevention of childhood obesity:

**Self-Reflection:** Journaling encourages children to reflect on their habits, fostering greater self-awareness and a deeper understanding of their choices.

**Mindful Choices:** Recording activities, food choices, and emotions helps children make more mindful decisions about their health and well-being.

**Empowerment:** By taking an active role in tracking their activities and choices, children gain a sense of control over their health journey.

**Behavior Patterns:** Journaling reveals patterns, allowing children to identify trends in their activities, food choices, and emotions.

**Emotional Well-Being:** The practice of journaling provides an outlet for children to express their thoughts and feelings, promoting emotional health.

## Writing a Journey to Wellness

In the world of "Wellness Journaling," the act of writing becomes a voyage of self-discovery and transformation. This strategy empowers children to navigate their well-being journey with intention, as they observe, learn, and make decisions that align with their health goals. As they put pen to paper, they craft not just words but a narrative of empowerment, growth, and a commitment to living a life of vitality and mindful choices.

# Strategy 15: Nature Scavenger Hunts

In the embrace of nature's playground, the "Nature Scavenger Hunts" strategy unfolds as an exhilarating way to spark children's curiosity while promoting outdoor exploration and movement. By organizing scavenger hunts that lead children on journeys of discovery, this approach transforms outdoor spaces into realms of adventure, physical activity, and wonder.

**Nature as the Ultimate Playground:** Imagine a world where every outdoor space becomes a treasure trove of hidden wonders waiting to be discovered. "Nature Scavenger Hunts" invite children to engage with their environment in a whole new way, as they search for clues, discover hidden treasures, and immerse themselves in the beauty of the natural world.

## Crafting Outdoor Quests

At the heart of this strategy lies the art of designing scavenger hunts that encourage movement, exploration, and connection with nature. Picture children eagerly exploring a park, garden, or forest, armed with lists of items to find and observe. These items could range from leaves, rocks, and flowers to animal tracks, bird nests, and interesting textures.

**Example: The Eco-Explorer Hunt:** Imagine a "Eco-Explorer Hunt" set in a local park. Children are given a list of natural items to find, such as a pinecone, a feather, a smooth stone, and a leaf of a certain color. As they explore, they engage in physical activity by walking, bending, and reaching to collect their treasures. Along the way, they discover the wonders of their environment and foster a connection with the natural world.

## Promoting Outdoor Adventure and Preventing Obesity

"Nature Scavenger Hunts" offer numerous advantages in the realm of childhood obesity prevention:

**Physical Exploration:** Children engage in physical activity as they move, walk, and explore outdoor spaces in search of clues and items.

**Nature Connection:** Scavenger hunts promote a connection with nature, nurturing a sense of wonder and appreciation for the outdoors.

**Imagination and Creativity:** Children's creativity is ignited as they use their imagination to hunt for items and solve clues.

**Positive Associations:** Outdoor adventure becomes associated with excitement, movement, and a sense of achievement.

**Family Bonding:** Scavenger hunts can become family activities, fostering shared moments of exploration and fun.

## Embarking on Nature's Quests

In the realm of "Nature Scavenger Hunts," children become adventurers, explorers, and eco-sleuths. This strategy invites them to step outside, observe their surroundings, and engage in physical activity while discovering the hidden treasures of nature. As they hunt, explore, and move through outdoor spaces, they cultivate not only a love for the natural world but also a deep appreciation for the joy of movement, curiosity, and the adventures that lead to a life rich with vitality and wonder.

# Strategy 16: Diverse Cultural Food Exploration

In the world of gastronomy and cultural diversity, the "Diverse Cultural Food Exploration" strategy unfolds as a flavorful and enlightening journey. By encouraging children to explore and appreciate the cuisine of different cultures, this approach transforms food into a bridge that connects them to the world while promoting healthy eating diversity.

**Cuisine as a Gateway to Culture**: Imagine a world where every meal is an opportunity to embark on a cultural adventure. "Diverse Cultural Food Exploration" invites children to venture beyond their culinary comfort zones, discovering the rich tapestry of flavors, ingredients, and traditions that different cultures offer.

## Embarking on Flavorful Expeditions

At the heart of this strategy lies the adventure of discovering and preparing foods from around the world. Picture children learning about different countries, their culinary traditions, and the key ingredients that define their cuisine. They explore recipes, try new ingredients, and participate in preparing dishes that showcase the flavors of diverse cultures.

**Example: The Global Tasting Tour:** Imagine a "Global Tasting Tour" where children explore a new country's cuisine each week. They learn about the ingredients, cooking techniques, and cultural significance of dishes from that country. They may prepare sushi from Japan, tacos from Mexico, curry from India, or pasta from Italy. Through hands-on cooking experiences, they learn to appreciate the balance of flavors, textures, and nutrition that different cuisines offer.

## Promoting Cultural Appreciation and Preventing Obesity

"Diverse Cultural Food Exploration" offers a range of benefits in the realm of childhood obesity prevention:

**Nutritional Diversity:** Exploring diverse cuisines introduces children to a wide variety of nutrient-rich ingredients and encourages a balanced diet.

**Cultural Awareness:** Learning about different cultures fosters appreciation, empathy, and a sense of global interconnectedness.

**Expanded Palate**: Trying new foods broadens children's palates and reduces the risk of food monotony, making them more open to healthier options.

**Educational Engagement:** This strategy combines food, geography, history, and cultural studies, offering a holistic learning experience.

**Positive Attitudes:** Encountering new flavors in a positive and supportive environment nurtures a positive attitude toward nutritious eating.

## Culinary Journeys of Discovery

In the realm of "Diverse Cultural Food Exploration," children become culinary explorers, cultural ambassadors, and global food enthusiasts. This strategy invites them to embark on flavorful journeys that celebrate diversity, encourage healthy eating habits, and enrich their understanding of the world's culinary treasures. As they savor global flavors, they also cultivate a love for the art of cooking, a curiosity for different cultures, and a lifelong commitment to embracing nutritious, diverse, and delicious foods.

# Strategy 17: Obstacle Course Playgrounds

In the realm of play and physicality, the "Obstacle Course Playgrounds" strategy emerges as an innovative approach that transforms local playgrounds into dynamic spaces of adventure and creative physical activity. By designing mini obstacle courses, this strategy invites children to engage in active play, conquer challenges, and experience the thrill of movement in a playful setting.

**Playgrounds as Adventure Zones:** Imagine a playground that becomes a realm of exploration, where every structure is a stepping stone in a thrilling obstacle course. "Obstacle Course Playgrounds" offer children an exciting twist on traditional playtime, as they navigate, jump, crawl, and climb their way through a series of creative challenges.

## Crafting Playful Challenges

At the heart of this strategy lies the art of designing obstacle courses that engage children's imagination and encourage physical movement. Picture children navigating a series of tasks that involve climbing up rope nets, crawling through tunnels, hopping on stepping stones, balancing on beams, and leaping over obstacles.

**Example: The Playground Adventure Quest:** Imagine a "Playground Adventure Quest" where children embark on a mission to complete a series of challenges. They start by crawling through a tunnel, then climb up a net structure, balance on a beam, jump from one platform to another, and finish by sliding down a slide. As they conquer each challenge, they engage in a full-body workout that blends fun with physical activity.

## Promoting Active Play and Preventing Obesity

"Obstacle Course Playgrounds" offer numerous benefits in the prevention of childhood obesity:

**Whole-Body Movement**: Obstacle courses engage different muscle groups and promote a full range of movements, from climbing and crawling to jumping and balancing.

**Active Imagination:** Creative challenges ignite children's imagination, turning physical activity into an adventure-driven experience.

**Motor Skills:** Obstacle courses enhance motor skills, coordination, and balance as children navigate through various challenges.

**Confidence Building:** Conquering challenges and completing courses fosters a sense of accomplishment and boosts self-confidence.

**Playful Engagement:** Children are drawn to playgrounds for active play, fostering a habit of enjoying movement and outdoor activities.

## Playful Exploration and Movement Mastery

In the realm of "Obstacle Course Playgrounds," children become adventurers, explorers, and movement masters. This strategy transforms traditional playgrounds into captivating landscapes of physical challenges and imaginative play. As they navigate, climb, and conquer obstacles, they cultivate not only physical strength but also a sense of excitement, creativity, and a lifelong love for the exhilarating blend of movement and play.

# Strategy 18: Family Nutrition Quizzes

In the realm of shared knowledge and connection, the "Family Nutrition Quizzes" strategy emerges as a delightful approach that brings families together to learn and bond while exploring the world of nutrition. By engaging in fun and educational quizzes, this strategy transforms learning about nutrition facts into an interactive and enriching experience.

**Quizzes as Family Adventures:** Imagine a world where learning becomes a family adventure, and nutritional facts are the treasure to be discovered. "Family Nutrition Quizzes" encourage families to gather, explore, and engage in friendly competition as they test their knowledge of healthy eating.

## Creating Educational Challenges

At the heart of this strategy lies the art of crafting quizzes that cover a range of nutritional topics. Picture families gathering around the table, taking turns to answer questions about food groups, portion sizes, vitamins, minerals, and the nutritional benefits of various foods.

**Example: The Nutritional Treasure Hunt:** Imagine a "Nutritional Treasure Hunt" quiz where family members answer questions about the nutritional value of different foods. Questions could include identifying which foods are good sources of specific nutrients, understanding portion control, and recognizing the benefits of whole grains, fruits, and vegetables. The family works together to uncover the "treasure" of knowledge about healthy eating.

## Promoting Learning and Connection and Preventing Obesity

"Family Nutrition Quizzes" offer a range of advantages in the realm of childhood obesity prevention:

**Educational Engagement:** Quizzes transform learning about nutrition into an interactive and enjoyable experience for the whole family.

**Shared Knowledge:** Families learn together, fostering open conversations about nutrition and healthy choices.

**Positive Associations:** Nutritional learning becomes associated with fun, bonding, and collaborative exploration.

**Mindful Eating:** Quizzes encourage awareness of nutritional facts, influencing mindful food choices.

**Quality Time:** Families bond while engaging in an activity that promotes wellness and healthy habits.

## Quiz-Time Adventures in Learning

In the realm of "Family Nutrition Quizzes," mealtimes and family gatherings become opportunities for shared exploration and learning. This strategy invites families to come together, laugh, learn, and bond as they embark on an adventure of nutritional knowledge. As they uncover facts, celebrate successes, and engage in playful competition, they cultivate not only their understanding of nutrition but also a lasting connection rooted in the joy of learning and well-being.

# Strategy 19: Interactive Cooking Shows

In the world of culinary exploration and healthy living, the "Interactive Cooking Shows" strategy emerges as a flavorful and educational approach that brings the excitement of cooking into the home. By watching cooking shows that focus on healthy recipes and techniques, this strategy transforms meal preparation into a delightful, interactive, and enriching experience.

**Cooking Shows as Home Culinary Adventures:** Imagine a world where the kitchen becomes a stage for culinary creativity, and cooking shows become a source of inspiration. "Interactive Cooking Shows" invite families to gather in the kitchen, explore new recipes, and engage in cooking together while learning about nutritious ingredients and techniques.

## Turning Screens into Kitchens

At the heart of this strategy lies the art of choosing and watching cooking shows that emphasize healthy cooking. Picture families tuning in to shows that feature chefs demonstrating step-by-step recipes, offering tips on ingredient selection, portion control, and cooking methods that support a balanced diet.

**Example: The Family MasterChef Experience:** Imagine a "Family MasterChef Experience" where families watch a cooking show together. They follow along as the chef prepares a delicious, nutritious meal. The show encourages interactivity by pausing at key moments to explain cooking techniques, discuss the benefits of certain ingredients, and answer questions from viewers. Families can replicate the recipe in their own kitchen, creating a shared culinary adventure.

## Promoting Culinary Learning and Preventing Obesity

"Interactive Cooking Shows" offer numerous advantages in the realm of childhood obesity prevention:

**Culinary Education:** Cooking shows provide valuable lessons about nutrition, ingredient selection, cooking techniques, and portion sizes.

**Healthy Inspiration:** Families are inspired to try new recipes and explore healthier cooking methods and ingredient choices.

**Interactive Learning:** Pause-and-play features engage families in discussions and practical demonstrations, enhancing learning.

**Shared Experience:** Cooking shows become a platform for families to bond while cooking, learning, and enjoying nutritious meals.

**Skill Development:** Family members, especially children, learn culinary skills that empower them to make healthier meals on their own.

## Cooking Together, Learning Together

In the realm of "Interactive Cooking Shows," the kitchen becomes a haven of learning, bonding, and healthy experimentation. This strategy encourages families to gather, cook, and learn while watching cooking shows that prioritize health and nutrition. As they chop, stir, and savor the results of their efforts, families cultivate not only a love for cooking but also a deeper understanding of how nutritious choices and culinary techniques contribute to a vibrant and well-balanced lifestyle.

# Strategy 20: Fitness Charades

In the realm of physical activity and entertainment, the "Fitness Charades" strategy is a playful approach that combines movement and guessing games. By playing charades with fitness-themed actions, this strategy transforms physical activity into a joyful and interactive experience that gets everyone moving, guessing, and laughing.

**Charades as Active Playtime:** Imagine a world where movement becomes a form of creative expression, and guessing games inspire laughter and camaraderie. "Fitness Charades" encourages families and friends to gather, take turns, and immerse themselves in a game that blends physical activity with the joy of playful interaction.

## Infusing Movement with Fun

At the heart of this strategy lies the art of incorporating fitness-related actions into the classic game of charades. Picture players performing actions like jumping jacks, hula hooping, yoga poses, bicycle pedaling, and more, while others guess the activity based on their movements.

**Example: The Active Charades Extravaganza:** Imagine an "Active Charades Extravaganza" where players draw fitness-related actions from a hat. One player acts out the action without speaking, while the others guess the activity. As they mimic activities like skipping rope, pretending to swim, or imitating a tree pose, they engage in a delightful and hilarious spectacle of movement.

## Promoting Playful Movement and Preventing Obesity

"Fitness Charades" offer a range of benefits in the realm of childhood obesity prevention:

**Physical Engagement:** The game encourages players to perform a variety of physical activities, promoting movement and exercise.

**Social Interaction:** Charades foster communication, collaboration, and bonding as players interact and guess together.

**Joyful Atmosphere:** Laughter and entertainment make physical activity enjoyable, encouraging regular participation.

**Creative Expression:** Players use their bodies to convey actions, fostering creativity and physical expression.

**Family and Friends Bonding:** The game becomes a platform for shared moments and a common goal of having fun while being active.

## Guess, Act, Move, Repeat

In the realm of "Fitness Charades," players become actors, guessers, and movement enthusiasts all at once. This strategy transforms physical activity into a game of fun and laughter, creating an environment where fitness is celebrated as an enjoyable and social endeavor. As they jump, stretch, and mimic their way through the game, players cultivate not only their bodies but also their spirits, forming lasting memories of active play and shared joy.

# Strategy 21: Cooking Science Experiments

In the realm of culinary curiosity and scientific discovery, the "Cooking Science Experiments" strategy emerges as a captivating approach that transforms the kitchen into a laboratory of nutritional exploration. By conducting cooking experiments that reveal how different foods affect the body, this strategy engages children in hands-on learning that intertwines science with the art of cooking.

**Culinary Lab Adventures:** Imagine a world where the kitchen becomes a place of scientific inquiry, where pots and pans become instruments of exploration. "Cooking Science

Experiments" invite children to roll up their sleeves, don their aprons, and embark on a culinary journey that uncovers the fascinating ways in which foods interact with the body.

## Blending Nutrition and Experimentation

At the heart of this strategy lies the fusion of culinary creativity and scientific investigation. Picture children designing and conducting experiments that illustrate the impact of various nutrients on the body. They explore questions such as how different foods affect energy levels, digestion, and overall well-being.

**Example: The Energy-Fuel Experiment:** Imagine conducting an "Energy-Fuel Experiment" with children. They prepare two different types of breakfasts—one with a balanced combination of carbohydrates, proteins, and healthy fats, and another with mostly sugary foods. After consuming each breakfast, they measure their energy levels, focus, and attention throughout the morning. The experiment sparks a discussion about how different foods provide sustained energy and affect their cognitive performance.

## Promoting Scientific Inquiry and Preventing Obesity

"Cooking Science Experiments" offer a range of advantages in the realm of childhood obesity prevention:

**Hands-On Learning:** Experiments provide a tangible way for children to understand how foods impact their bodies.

**Scientific Curiosity:** Children engage in scientific thinking, forming hypotheses, conducting experiments, and drawing conclusions.

**Nutritional Literacy:** Experimentation fosters a deeper understanding of nutrients, their functions, and the importance of balanced eating.

**Mindful Choices:** Insights from experiments influence children's food choices, encouraging them to make healthier decisions.

**Empowerment:** Children become active participants in their health journey, equipped with knowledge about the foods they consume.

## Exploring Nutrition Through Playful Science

In the realm of "Cooking Science Experiments," the kitchen becomes a realm of exploration, where pots bubble with curiosity and pans sizzle with discovery. This strategy invites children to be culinary scientists, uncovering the mysteries of nutrition through hands-on experimentation. As they mix, measure, and observe, they cultivate not only an understanding of how food affects their bodies but also a lifelong love for the intersection of science, cooking, and well-being.

# Strategy 22: DIY Healthy Snack Creations

In the realm of culinary creativity and nutritional empowerment, the "DIY Healthy Snack Creations" strategy emerges as an empowering approach that puts children in charge of designing their own nutritious snack options. By engaging children in the process of selecting ingredients and crafting their own snacks, this strategy transforms snack time into an opportunity for creativity and mindful eating.

**Snack Creation as Personal Expression:** Imagine a world where snack time becomes a canvas for culinary expression, and children are the artists who craft their own edible masterpieces. "DIY Healthy Snack Creations" encourage children to make informed choices, experiment with flavors, and take pride in their culinary creations.

## Nurturing Nutritional Decision-Making

At the heart of this strategy lies the act of empowering children to make choices about the foods they consume. Picture children selecting from a variety of wholesome ingredients—such as fruits, vegetables, whole grains, nuts, and seeds—and using their creativity to assemble their own unique and delicious snacks.

**Example: The Snack Picasso Workshop:** Imagine hosting a "Snack Picasso Workshop" where children are presented with an array of ingredients and invited to design their own snacks. They might start with a base of whole grain crackers or yogurt, then add a variety of toppings like berries, sliced cucumbers, cheese cubes, and a sprinkle of seeds. The workshop encourages children to consider flavor combinations, textures, and nutritional value as they create their own edible artworks.

## Promoting Nutritional Empowerment and Preventing Obesity

"DIY Healthy Snack Creations" offer a range of advantages in the realm of childhood obesity prevention:

**Personal Choice:** Children actively participate in selecting ingredients, promoting a sense of ownership over their food choices.

**Nutritional Awareness:** Crafting their own snacks increases awareness of nutritional values and the benefits of various ingredients.

**Creative Engagement:** Snack creation becomes a platform for imaginative expression and experimentation with flavors.

**Mindful Eating:** Children take time to think about their snack components, fostering mindful eating habits.

**Positive Attitudes**: A sense of accomplishment and pride accompanies the enjoyment of self-made snacks, promoting a positive attitude toward nutritious eating.

## Crafting Nutritious Edible Delights

In the realm of "DIY Healthy Snack Creations," children become culinary architects, designers, and decision-makers. This strategy invites them to assemble, experiment, and explore flavors while making informed choices about their snacks. As they sprinkle, layer, and assemble their creations, they cultivate not only their palates but also their sense of ownership over their well-being and a lifelong love for culinary creativity and wholesome eating.

# Strategy 23: Animal Movement Imitation

In the realm of outdoor exploration and imaginative play, the "Animal Movement Imitation" strategy emerges as a captivating approach that combines the wonder of nature with physical activity and learning. By encouraging children to mimic the movements of animals during outdoor play, this strategy transforms the outdoors into a vibrant classroom of movement and discovery.

**Nature as a Movement Teacher:** Imagine a world where the natural world becomes a source of inspiration for movement and play. "Animal Movement Imitation" invites children to explore the outdoors, observe the movements of animals, and engage in physical activity that mirrors the graceful, energetic, and diverse ways animals navigate their environment.

## Merging Movement and Imagination

At the heart of this strategy lies the fusion of movement, imagination, and outdoor exploration. Picture children venturing into parks, gardens, or nature trails and imitating the movements of animals they encounter. They might leap like frogs, crawl like caterpillars, hop like rabbits, and balance like birds.

**Example: The Animal Movement Safari:** Imagine embarking on an "Animal Movement Safari" where children set out on a mission to imitate the movements of various animals they encounter. As they stroll, skip, hop, and flutter their way through the outdoors, they engage in a playful and educational adventure that connects them with the world of wildlife.

## Promoting Nature-Inspired Movement and Preventing Obesity

"Animal Movement Imitation" offers a range of benefits in the realm of childhood obesity prevention:

**Physical Activity**: Imitating animal movements encourages whole-body engagement, promoting physical exercise.

**Outdoor Exploration**: Children connect with nature, fostering a love for the outdoors and natural movement.

**Imagination and Creativity**: Imitating animal movements sparks imaginative play and creative expression.

**Educational Experience**: Children learn about animals and their unique ways of moving through real-life imitation.

**Positive Associations**: Movement becomes associated with fun and exploration, encouraging children to stay active.

## Nature-Inspired Play, Movement, and Learning

In the realm of "Animal Movement Imitation," children become explorers, observers, and imaginative movers. This strategy invites them to venture outdoors, engage in playful imitation, and experience the wonder of animal movements firsthand. As they hop, crawl, and flutter through the natural world, they cultivate not only physical agility but also a deep connection to nature, curiosity about animals, and a lifelong love for movement that is both joyous and educational.

# Strategy 24: DIY Fitness Equipment Crafts

In the realm of creativity and active living, the "DIY Fitness Equipment Crafts" strategy emerges as a hands-on approach that combines crafting with physical activity. By creating simple exercise equipment like jump ropes or yoga mats with children, this strategy transforms ordinary materials into tools for active play and movement.

**Crafting as Fitness Adventure:** Imagine a world where crafting becomes a gateway to physical activity and well-being, and everyday materials turn into fitness companions. "DIY Fitness Equipment Crafts" invite children to explore their creative side while also engaging in the process of crafting exercise tools they can use for active play.

## Crafting Movement Tools

At the heart of this strategy lies the art of using common materials to construct exercise equipment. Picture children working together to create jump ropes using ropes and handles, or crafting yoga mats from fabric and foam. These homemade tools become a tangible representation of their creative efforts and their commitment to physical fitness.

**Example: The DIY Fitness Craft Hour:** Imagine hosting a "DIY Fitness Craft Hour" where children gather to create exercise equipment. They might craft jump ropes from sturdy cords and handles, or assemble yoga mats using fabric and cushioning materials. After the crafting session, they get to test out their newly created fitness tools with active play.

## Promoting Creativity and Active Living

"DIY Fitness Equipment Crafts" offer a range of advantages in the realm of childhood obesity prevention:

**Hands-On Engagement:** Crafting engages children in a practical activity while also encouraging movement.

**Resourcefulness:** Children learn to repurpose materials and transform them into functional fitness tools.

**Ownership**: Crafting exercise equipment fosters a sense of ownership and pride over their creations.

**Active Play:** Homemade fitness tools inspire active play, encouraging movement and physical activity.

**Creative Expression:** Crafting nurtures creativity and resourcefulness, promoting a well-rounded approach to fitness.

## Crafting Health, Creativity, and Well-Being

In the realm of "DIY Fitness Equipment Crafts," children become inventors, creators, and active adventurers. This strategy encourages them to repurpose materials, craft their own fitness tools, and take ownership of their well-being. As they jump, stretch, and engage in active play using their homemade equipment, they cultivate not only physical strength but also a sense of creativity, resourcefulness, and a lifelong love for movement and active living.

# Strategy 25: Gratitude and Body Positivity Activities

In the realm of emotional well-being and self-acceptance, the "Gratitude and Body Positivity Activities" strategy emerges as a heartwarming and empowering approach that promotes a positive relationship with one's body. By engaging in activities that foster gratitude for the body and encourage self-acceptance, this strategy transforms the way children perceive themselves and their well-being.

**Activities for Inner Nurturing:** Imagine a world where self-love, gratitude, and body positivity are celebrated and cultivated. "Gratitude and Body Positivity Activities" invite children to embark on a journey of self-discovery and appreciation, acknowledging the uniqueness and beauty of their bodies.

## Shaping Positive Self-Image

At the heart of this strategy lies the art of engaging in activities that promote self-acceptance and body positivity. Picture children participating in activities that encourage them to focus on their strengths, appreciate their bodies' capabilities, and nurture a sense of gratitude for their well-being.

**Example: The Body Positivity Art Session**: Imagine hosting a "Body Positivity Art Session" where children create art that celebrates their bodies. They might draw self-portraits, create collages of images that represent their strengths, or write letters of gratitude to their bodies. These activities encourage reflection, self-expression, and the fostering of a positive self-image.

## Promoting Self-Love and Emotional Well-Being

"Gratitude and Body Positivity Activities" offer a range of benefits in the realm of childhood obesity prevention:

**Self-Appreciation:** Activities encourage children to focus on what their bodies can do and appreciate their uniqueness.

**Emotional Well-Being:** Fostering gratitude and body positivity supports children's mental and emotional health.

**Confidence Building:** Engaging in positive self-reflection nurtures self-esteem and self-confidence.

**Healthy Habits:** A positive self-image encourages children to make choices that support their overall well-being.

**Mind-Body Connection:** Activities promote awareness of the mind-body connection and the importance of self-care.

## Nurturing Inner Beauty and Positivity

In the realm of "Gratitude and Body Positivity Activities," children become champions of self-love, gratitude, and emotional well-being. This strategy empowers them to embrace their bodies, appreciate their strengths, and cultivate a positive self-image. As they engage in creative expression, self-reflection, and the celebration of their uniqueness, they foster not only a strong sense of self but also a lifelong commitment to nurturing their emotional and physical well-being.